BIBLE STORY

Some things about queen Esther and Mordecai

Sunday O. Aduragbemi

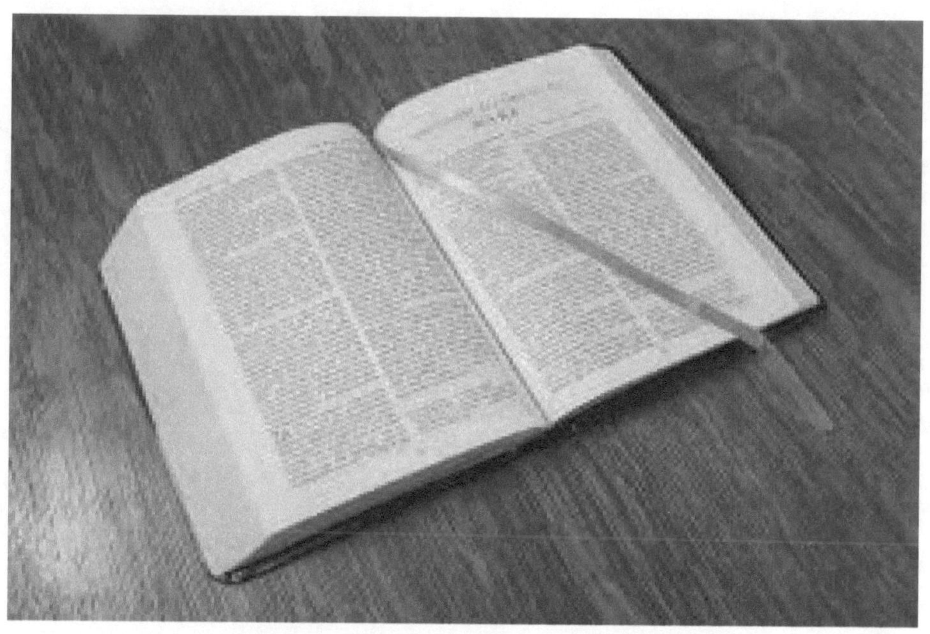

Copyright © 2019 by **Sunday O. Aduragbemi**

TABLE OF CONTENTS

INTRODUCTION

The story of Mordecai and Esther shows the power of the Almighty God in changing the present position of a person from a small level to a greater level. If only you can love, trust and obey the commandments of God in doing all that He wants from you, then there are lots of blessings that follows.

The Lord lifted up Esther right from the position of a slave and place her in the position of the queen and made her sat together with the great ones. God turns Mordecai from and ordinary servant and even a gatekeeper to the second-in-command to king Ahasuerus.

As young children, if only you can love God and work in total obedience to His ways, He is ready to bless you and make you great as you go into this story book.

CHAPTER ONE

Mordecai and Esther
Some few years earlier than ez'ra went to Jerusalem. Mor'decai and esther are the maximum important israelites inside the kingdom of Persia. Esther is the queen, and her cousin mor'de·cai is next to the king in strength. How did all this happen?

Esther's parents died when she turned into very small, and so mor'de·cai has raised her up.

A·has·u·e'rus, the king of persia, has a palace within the metropolis of shu'shan, and mor'de·cai is considered one of his servants. Well, sooner or later the king's spouse vash'ti does not obey him, so the king chooses a brand-new spouse to be his queen.

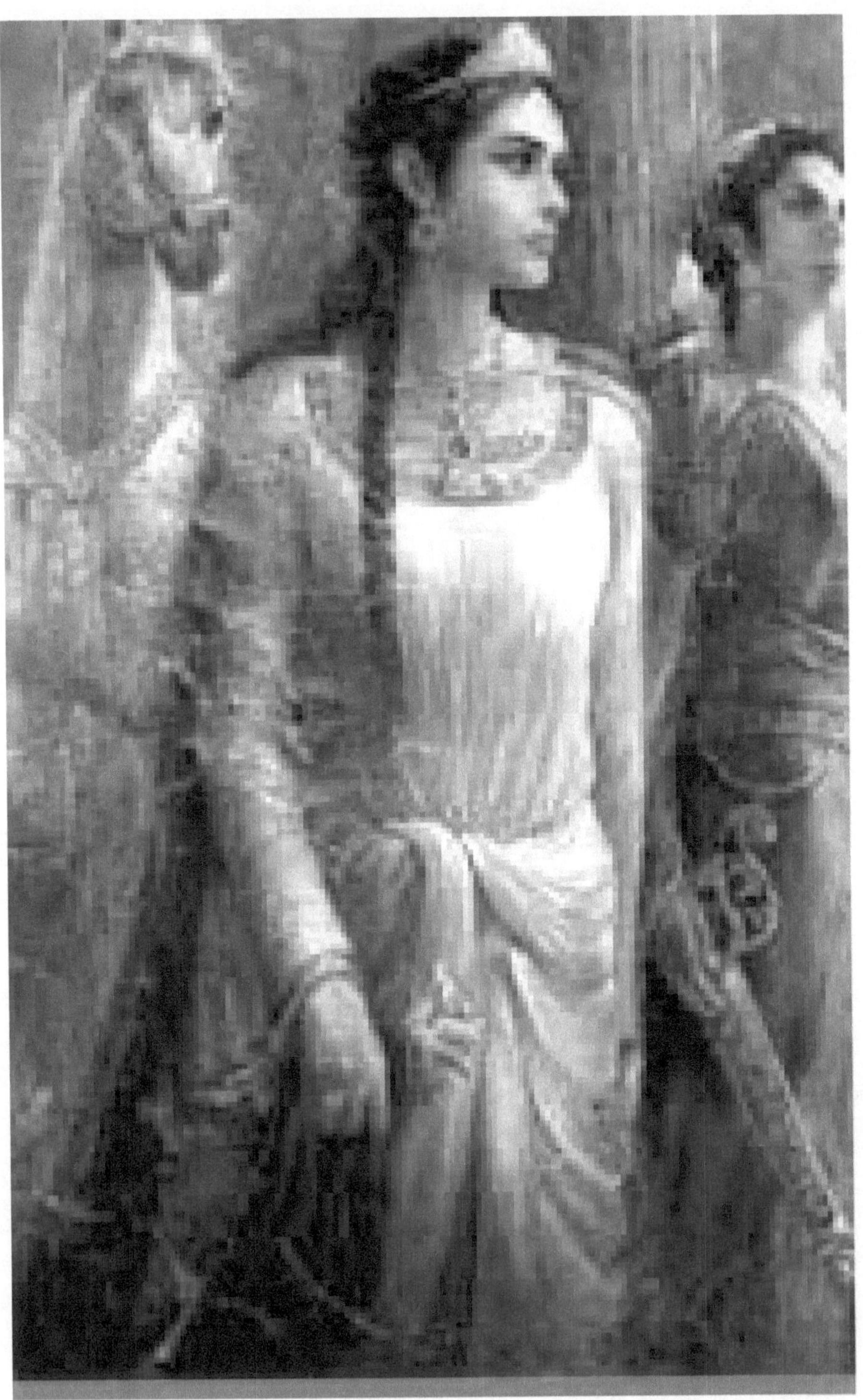

Who was the woman he chooses? Sure, it

was the young esther.

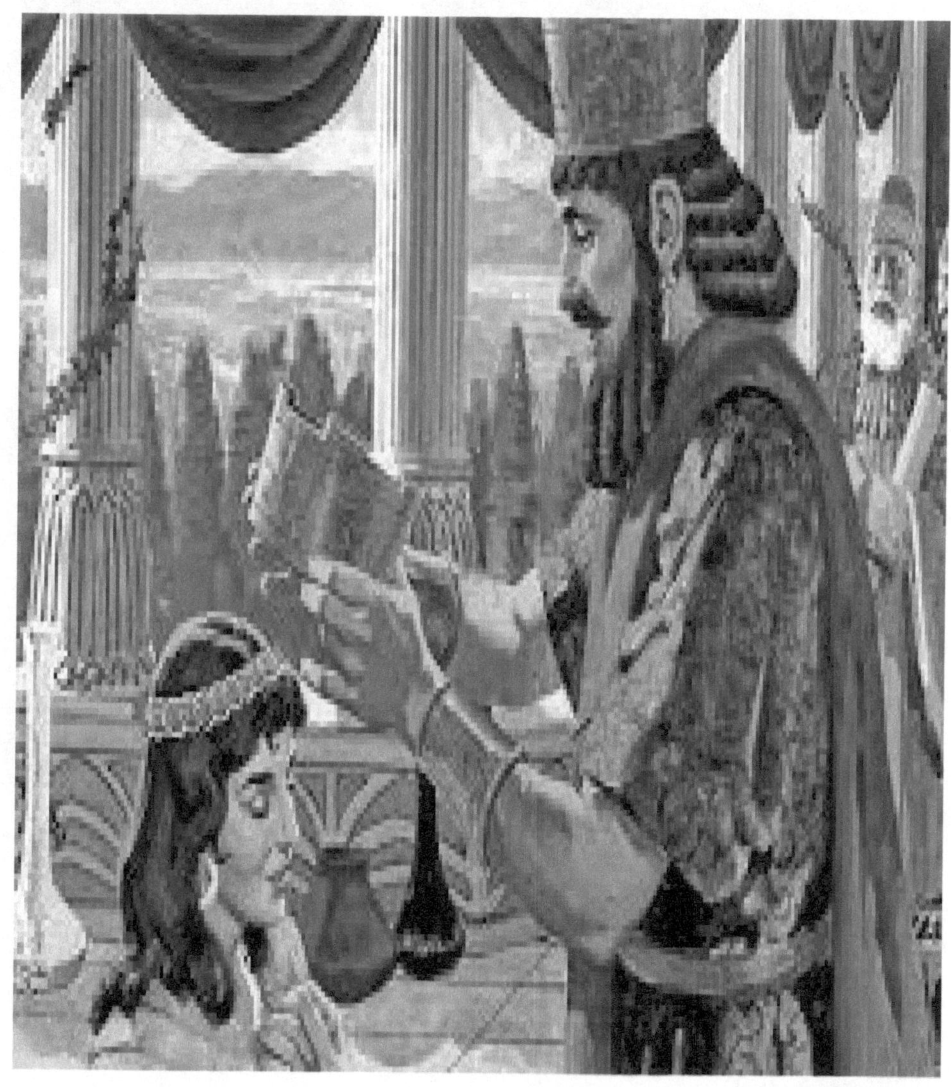

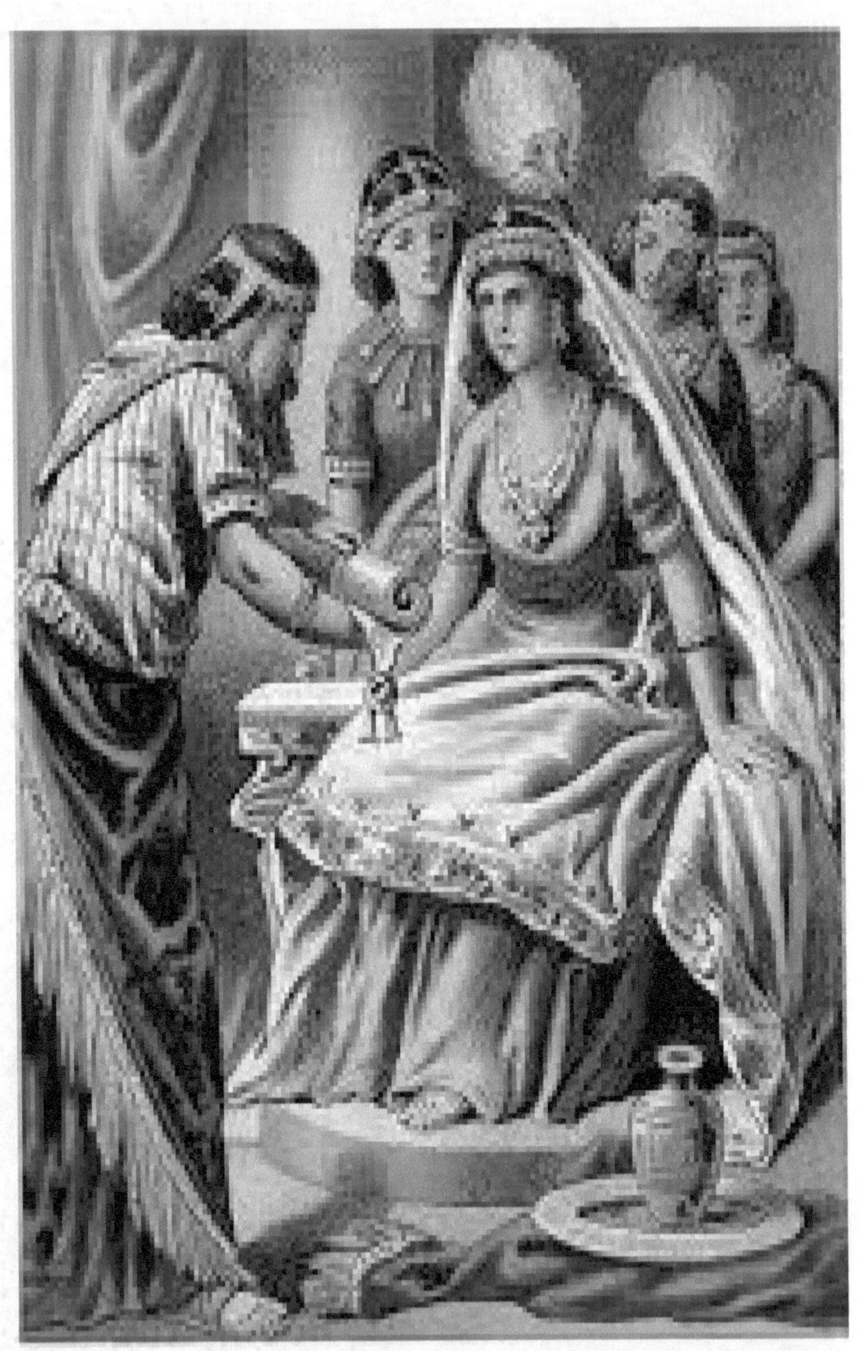

HATACH SHOWING ESTHER THE COPY OF THE WRITING OF THE DECREE.

CHAPTER TWO

Instructions from the existence of mordecai

1. Mordecai was ready to dis-satisfy himself for others to be satisfy.

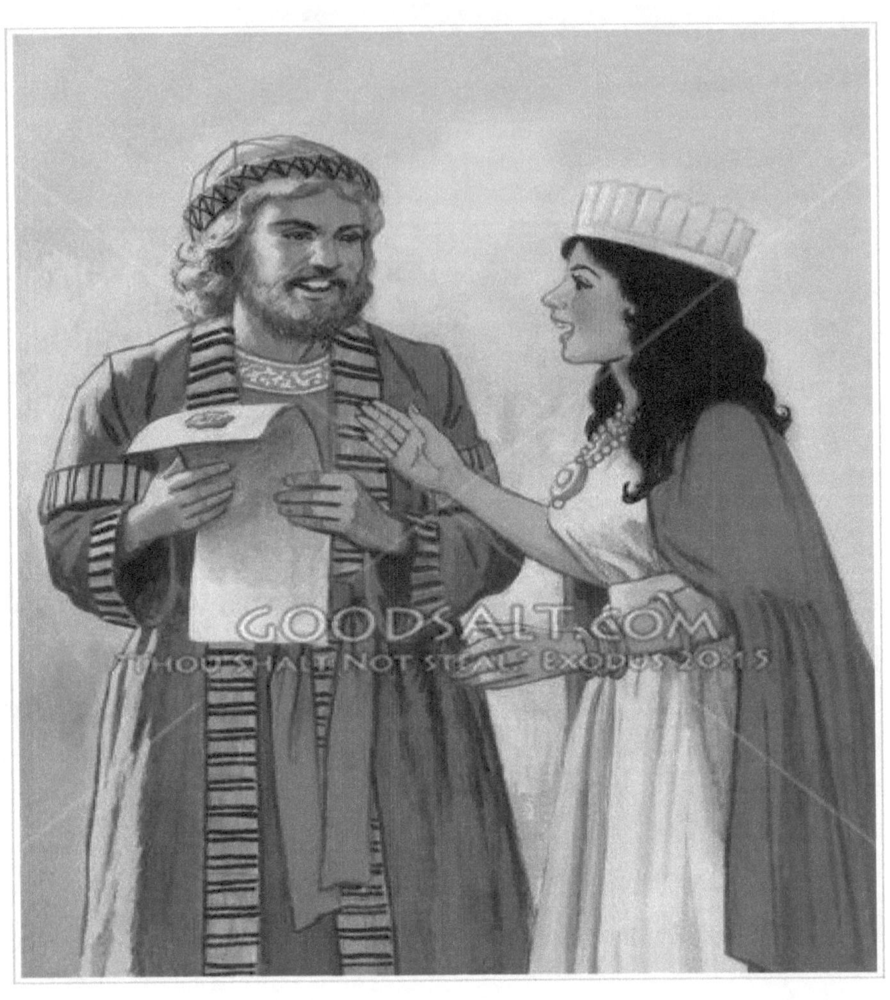

we can see that he changed into organized to

undertake his cousin as she had no parents…

so mordecai ought to have been willing to

step out and do what wasn't handy and

possibly wasn't comfy!

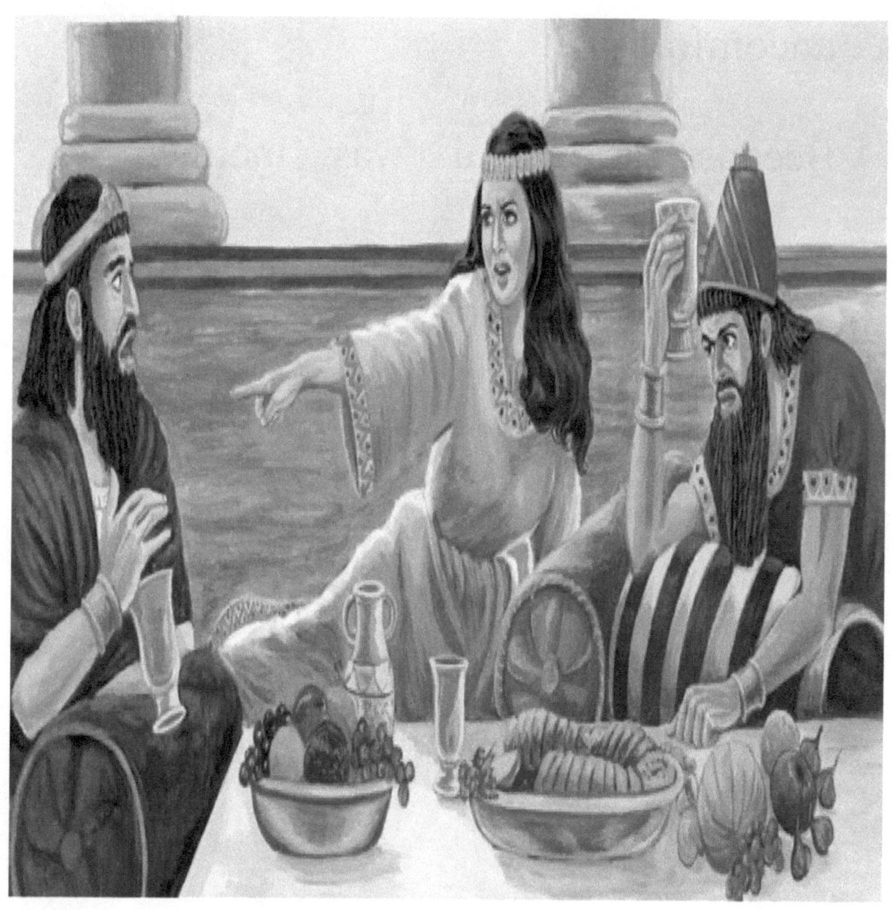

It reminded me that the leadership adventure is normally inconvenient and generally very uncomfortable!

Because mordecai was inclined to be inconvenienced and sense uncomfortable, he became able to store time.

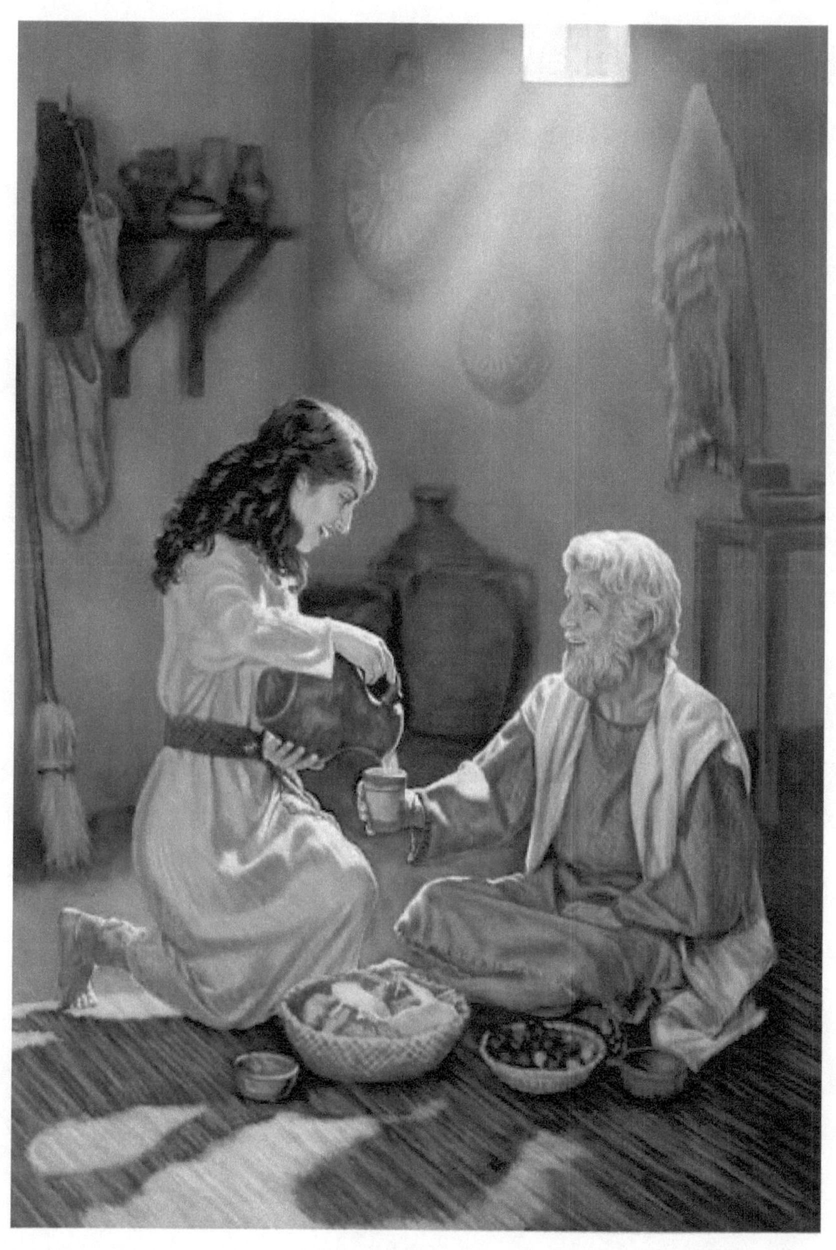

Are you willing to be inconvenienced and

uncomfortable?

2. He had excellent knowledge and loves to do what seems right at all time

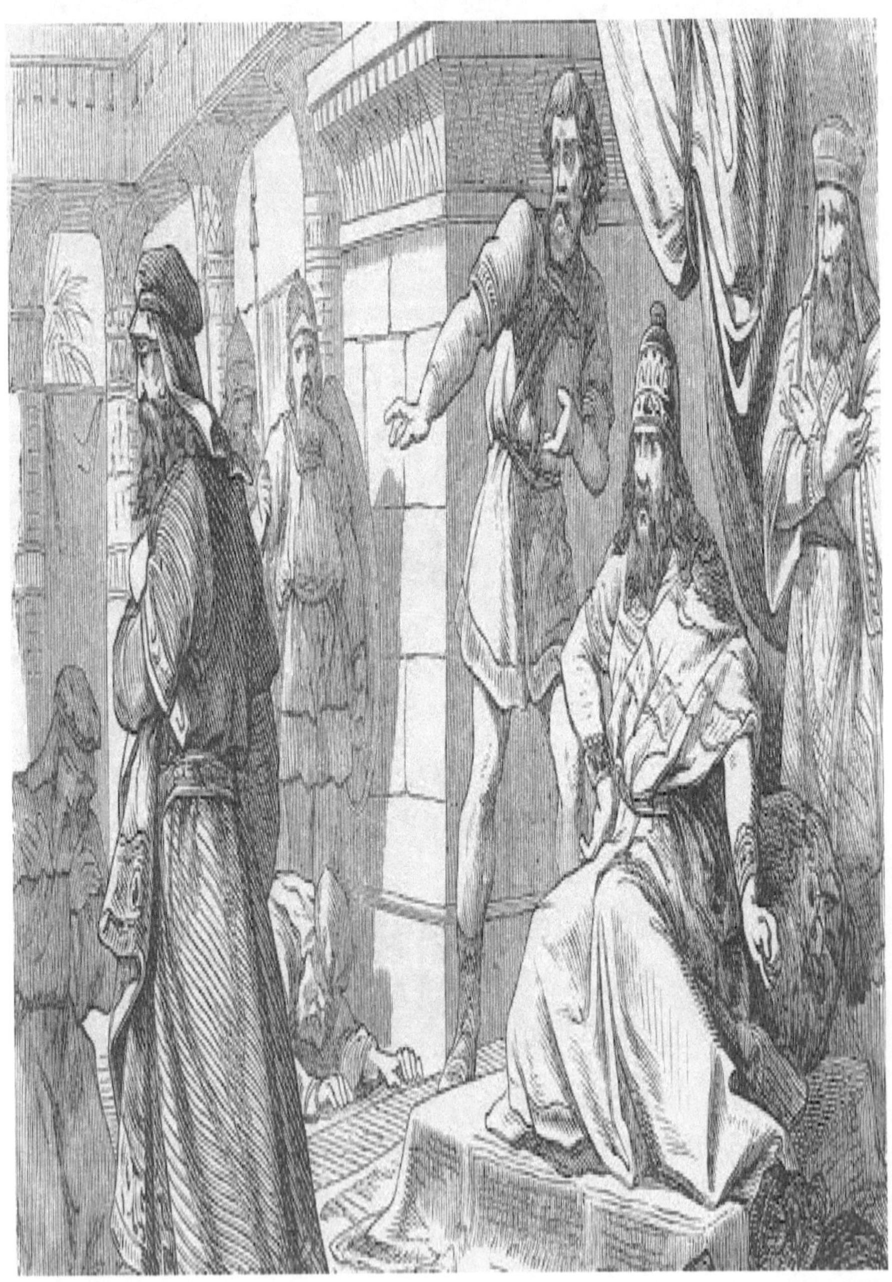

Mordecai told esther not to show her history after which while he heard the plot to assassinate the king, he changed into capable of becoming as clever as a serpent and gentle as a dove.

Genuine management constantly calls for awareness and integrity!

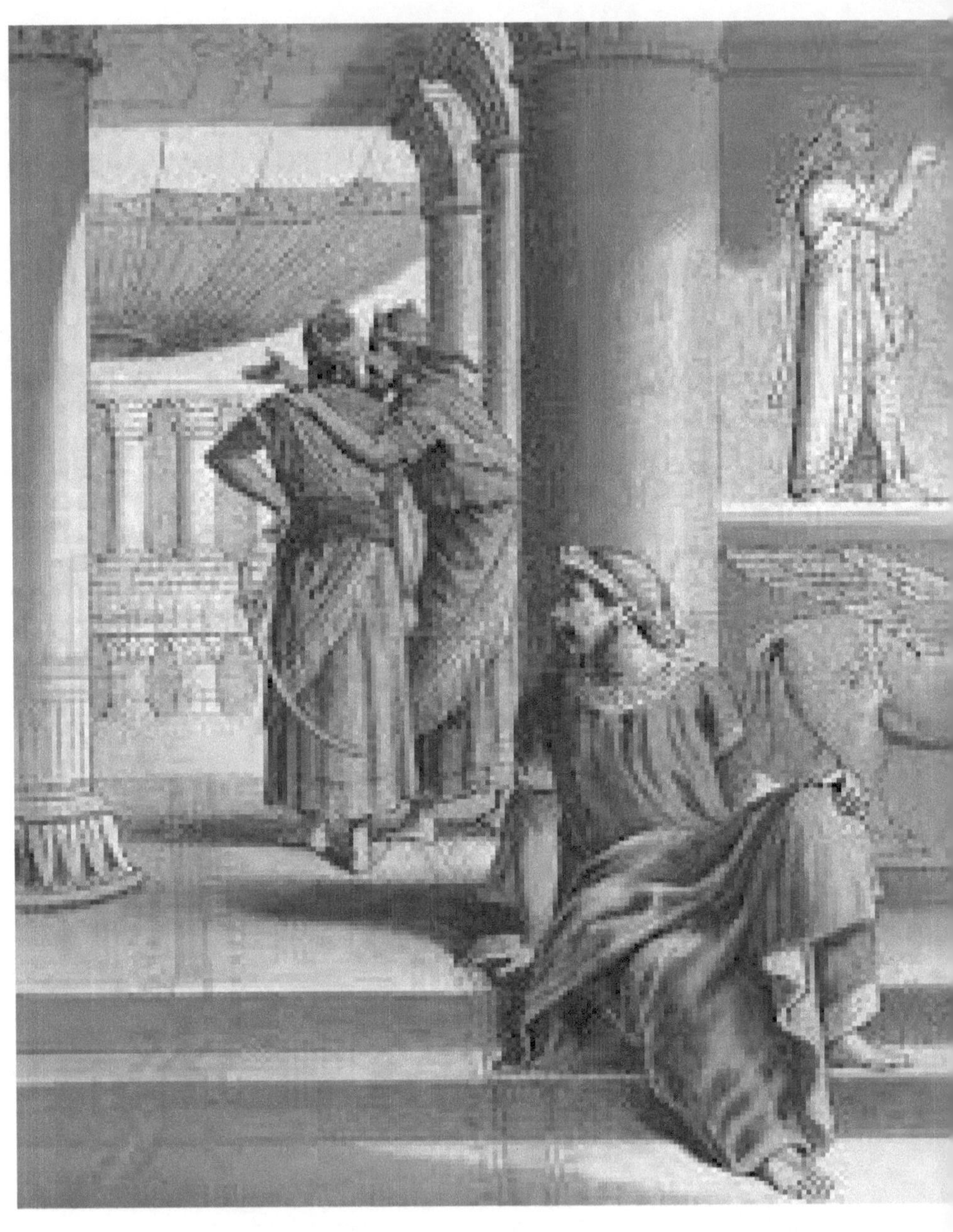

Mordecai said and did what become proper

honestly because it turned into proper!

3. He could not compromise

Chapter three tells us that mordecai might

no longer bow right down to haman!

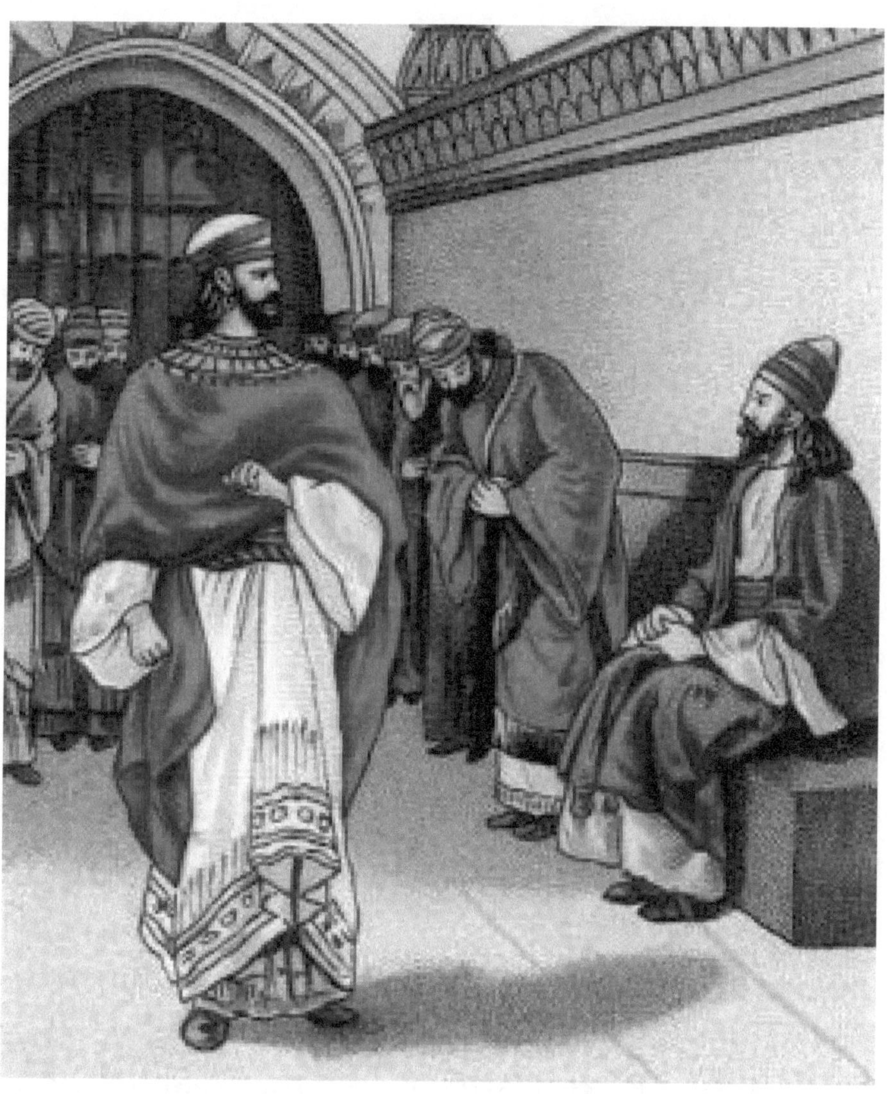

Do you spot this proud guy that human beings are bowing all the way down to? That is ha'man. He is a completely crucial man in persia. Ha'man wishes mor'de·cai, whom you can see sitting right here, to bow down to him also. However, mor'de·cai refused to do it. He doesn't assume it's far proper to bow all the way down to one of these terrible men.

Why, it does no longer say, however what it does reflect is that mordecai sees it unfit to bow down to the culture of the arena rather than the living God who created him.

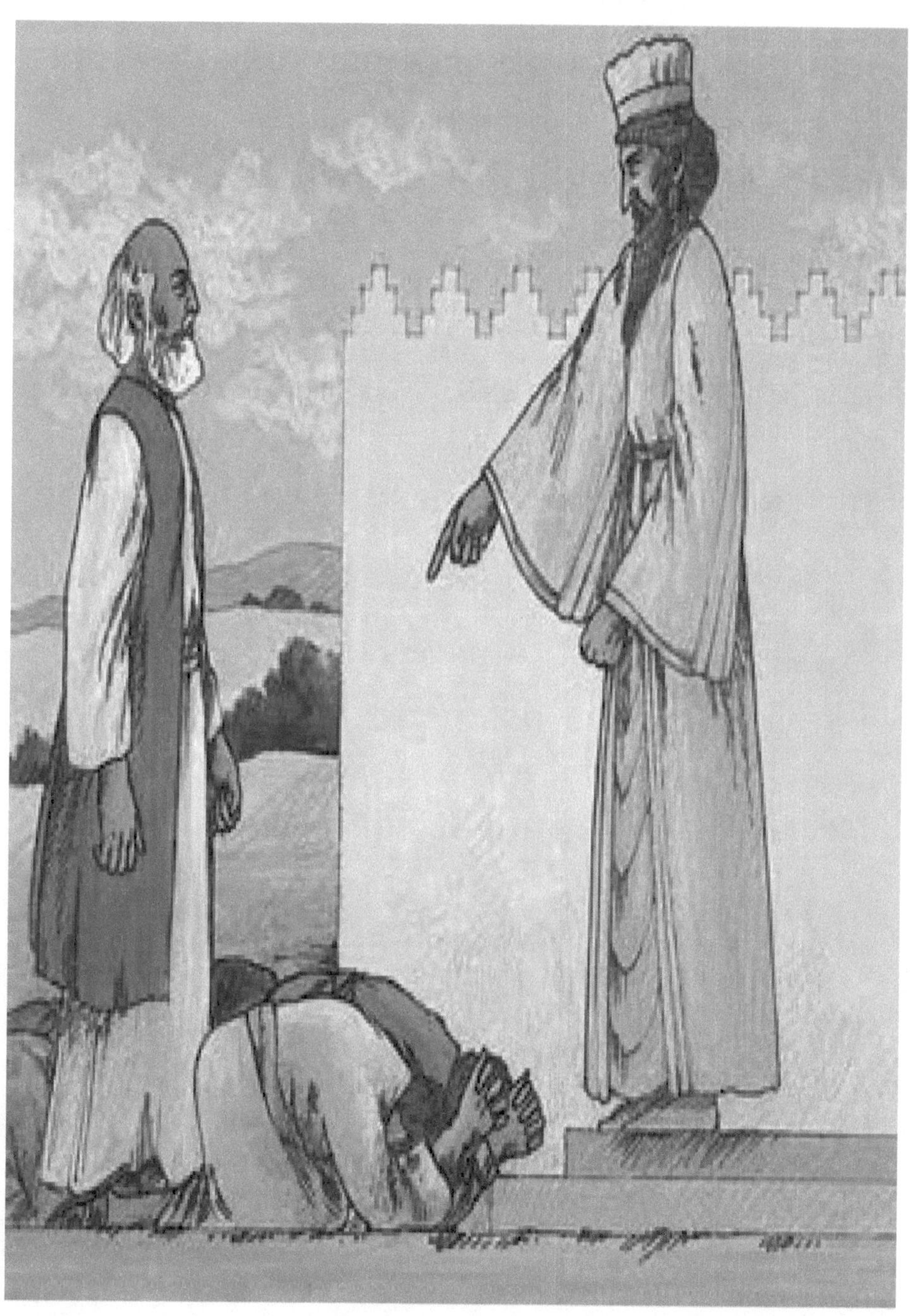

This makes Ha'man very irritated. And so that is what he does. Ha'man tells the king lies approximately the Israelites. 'they are horrific people who don't obey your legal guidelines,' he says. 'they have to be placed to death.' A·has·u·e'rus does not recognise that his wife Esther is an Israelite. So, he listens to Ha'man, and he has a regulation made that on a sure day all israelites are to be killed.

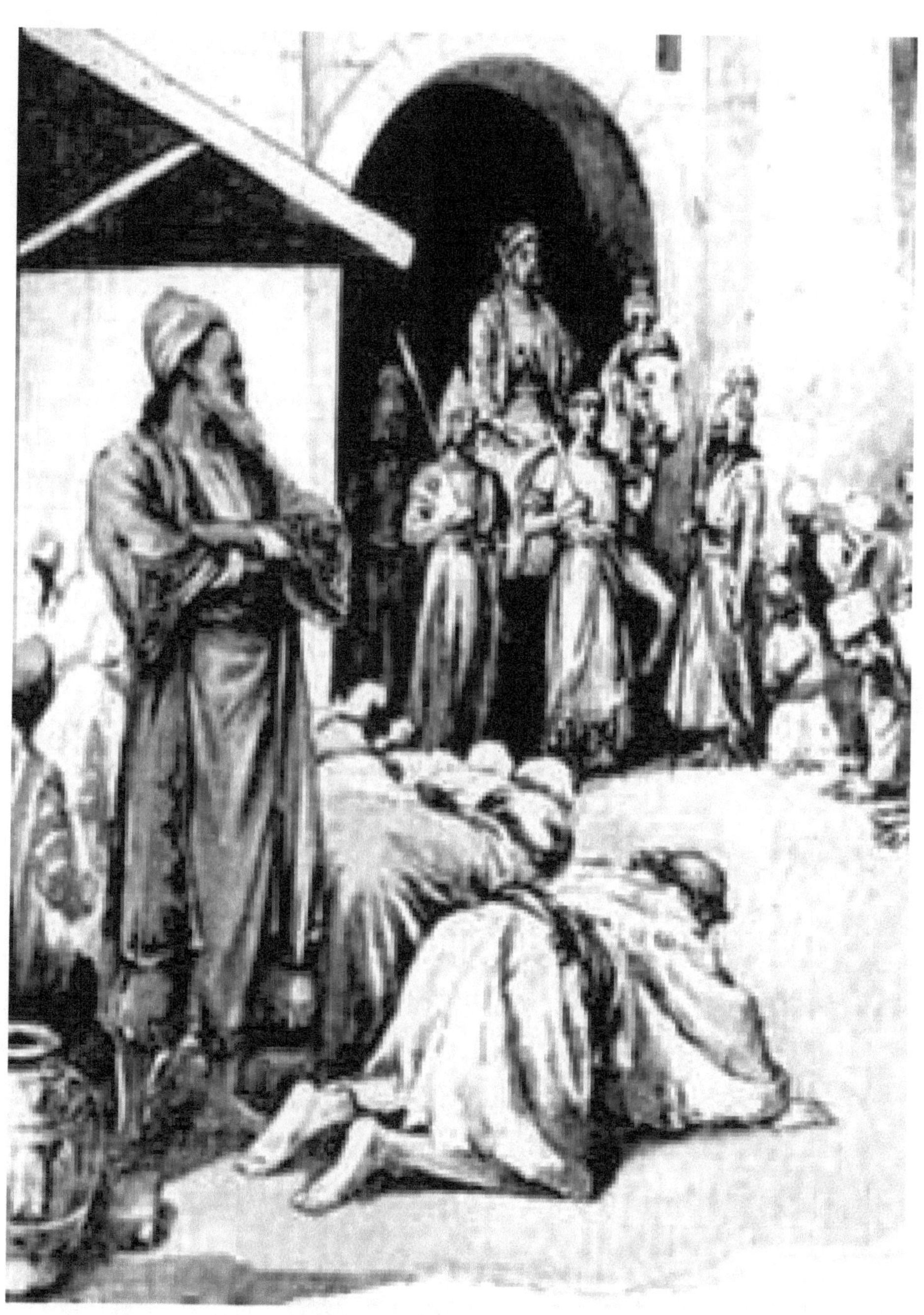

Thou shall not bow to any any other image except God.

There's no room for mediocrity or half off-hearted christianity! He changed into bought out, no compromise, 100% in, and I think powerful and fruitful management must be all in!

3. He become willing to risk what changed into dearest to him!

When Mor'de·cai hears about the regulation, he felt very dissatisfied. He sends a message to Esther: 'you have to inform the king, and beg him to deliver us.'

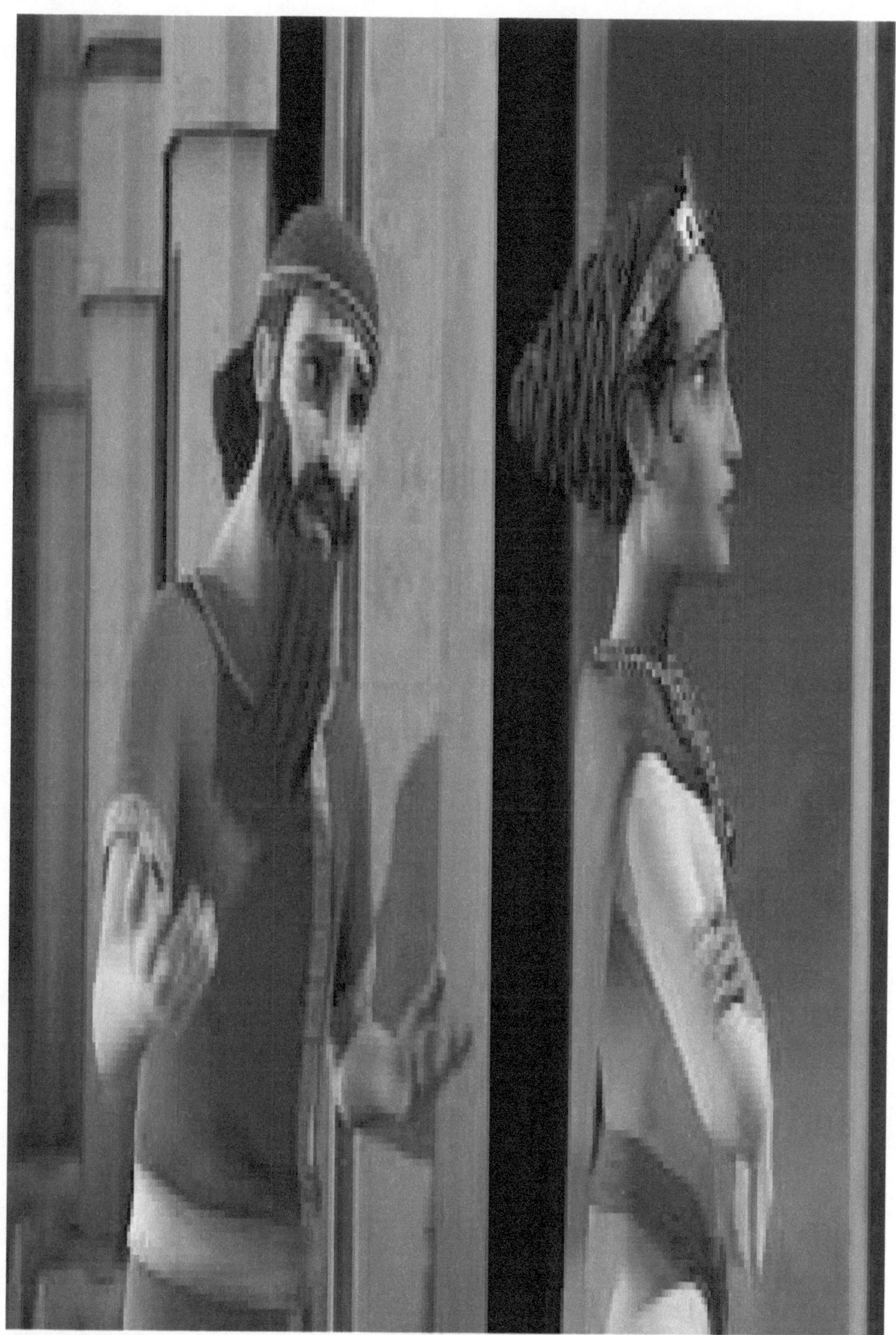

Hatach brought message from Mordecai to Queen Esther

In chapter four, it tells us that mordecai advocated esther to visit the king on behalf of the people.

This will have meant that he could potentially have misplaced esther, as this meant she turned in to danger her existence. But he should had been prepared to be counted to have paid the prize for the sake of others. What does the prize seem like for you? I'm hoping it isn't as extreme for you and I, as it was for mordecai, however let's never expect counting the prize to serve Jesus and our generation!

It's far against the law in persia to go closely

to the king except you are invited by him.

But Esther goes in with out being invited.

The king holds out his gold rod to her,

which means that that she isn't always to be

killed.

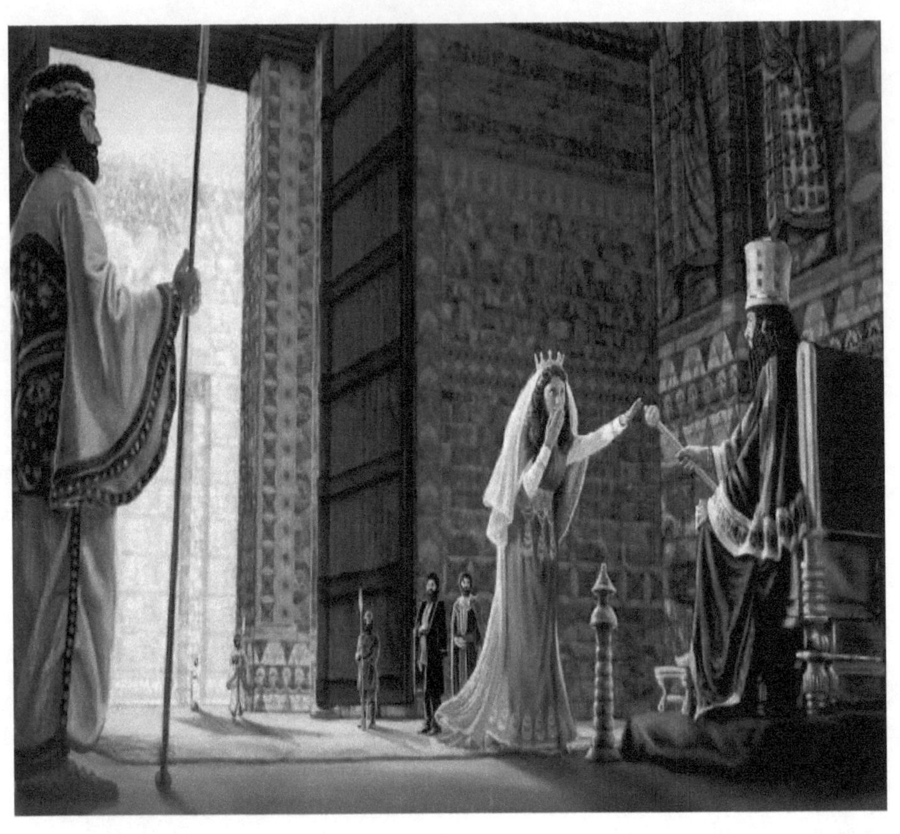

Esther risk her life for her people

Esther invites the king and ha'man to a huge meal. There the king asks Esther what was her wishes from him. Esther says that she can inform him if he and ha'man will come to another meal

tomorrow.

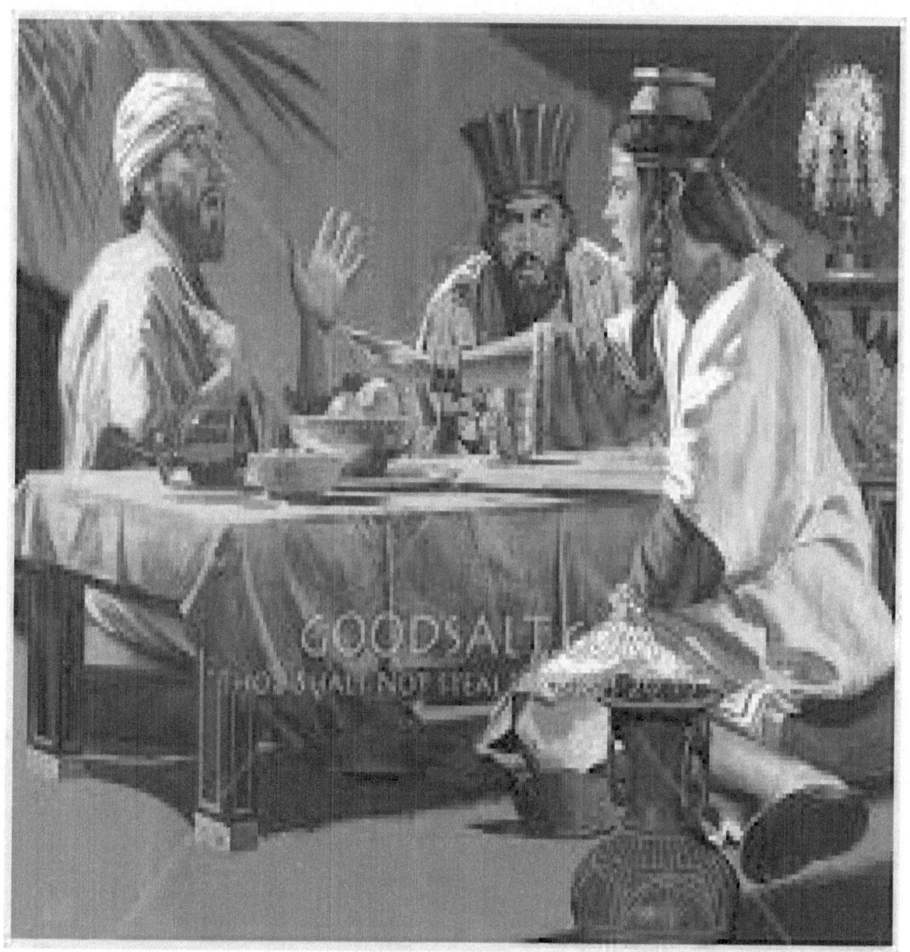

At that meal Esther tells the king: 'my people and I are to be killed.' the king is irritated. 'who dares to do the sort of component?' he asks.

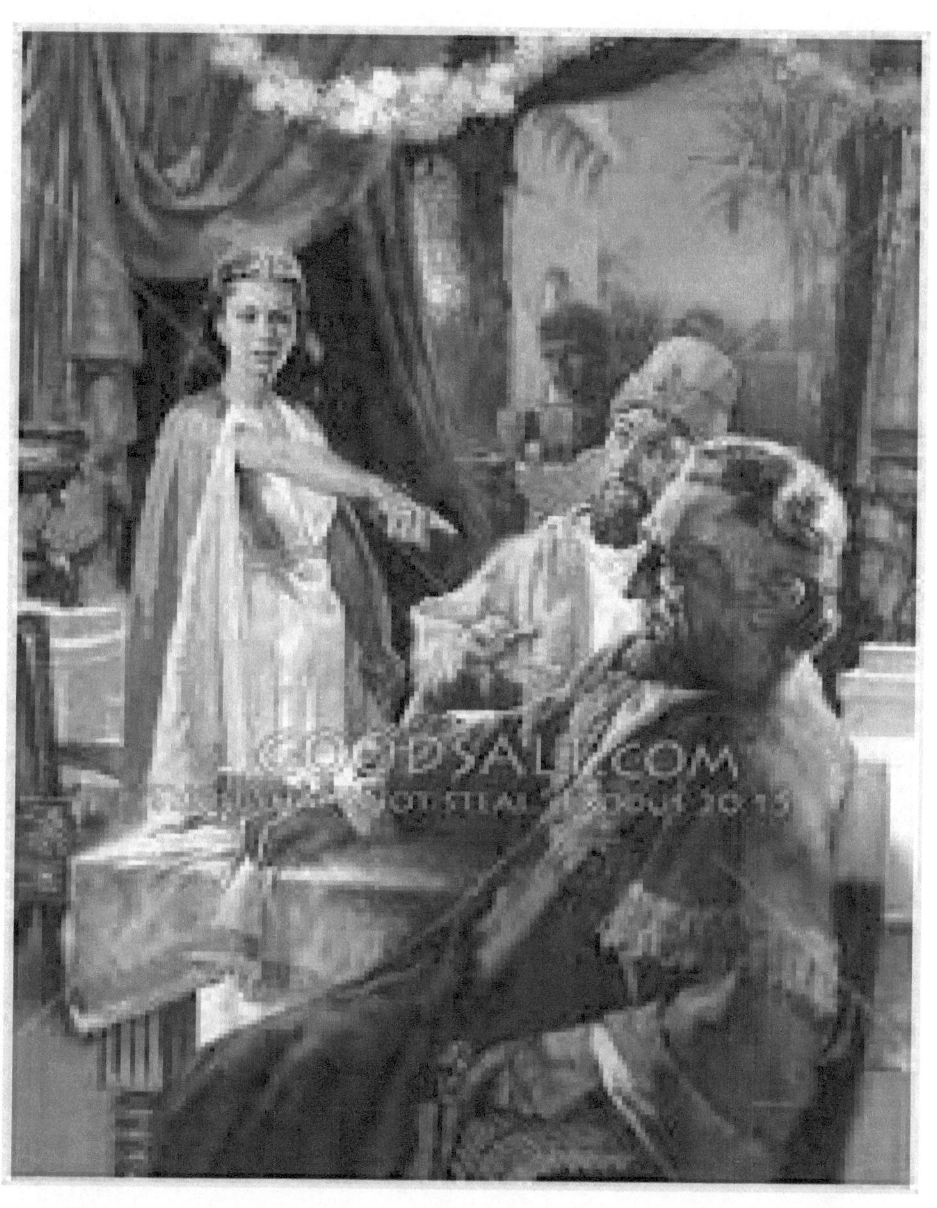

'The person, the enemy, is this terrible

Ha'man!' Esther says.

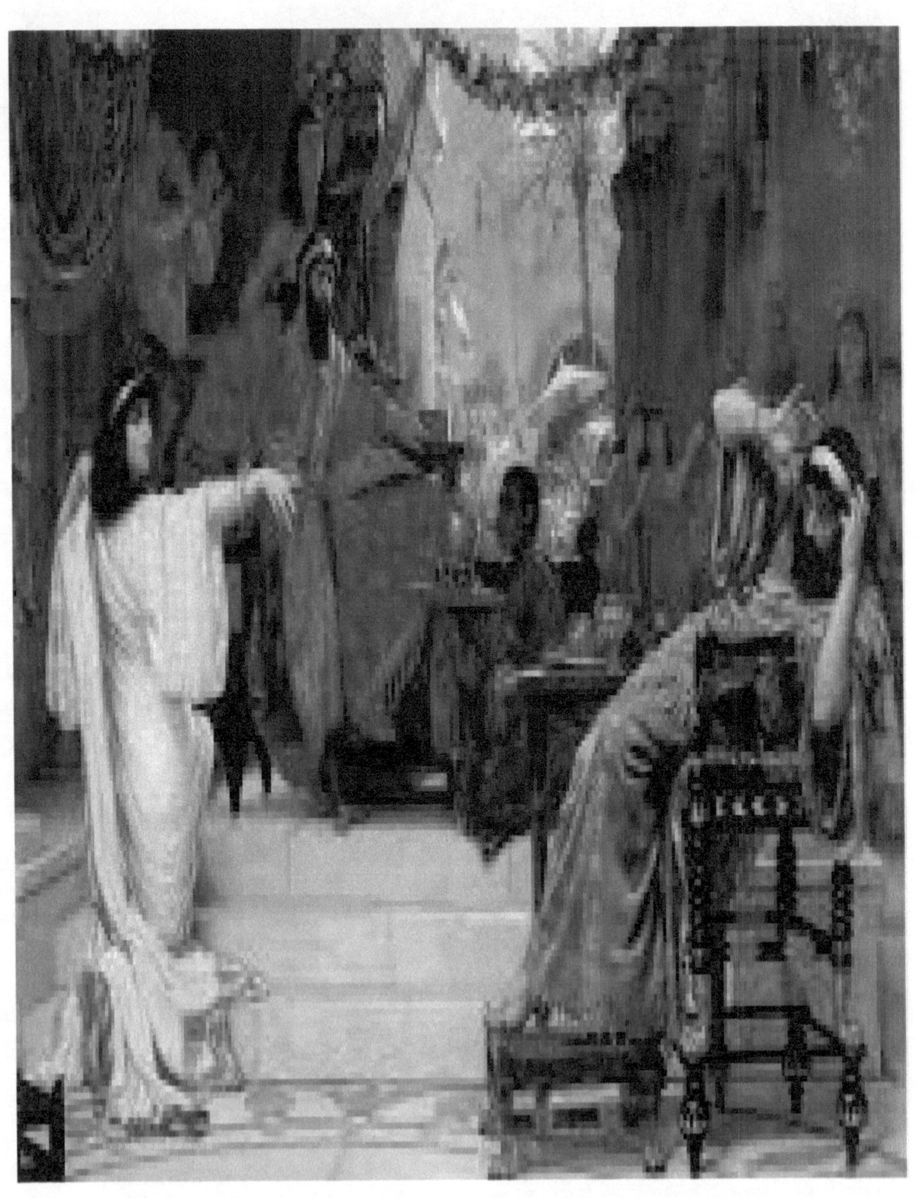

Now the king is indeed annoyed and then

instructed that Ha'man be killed.

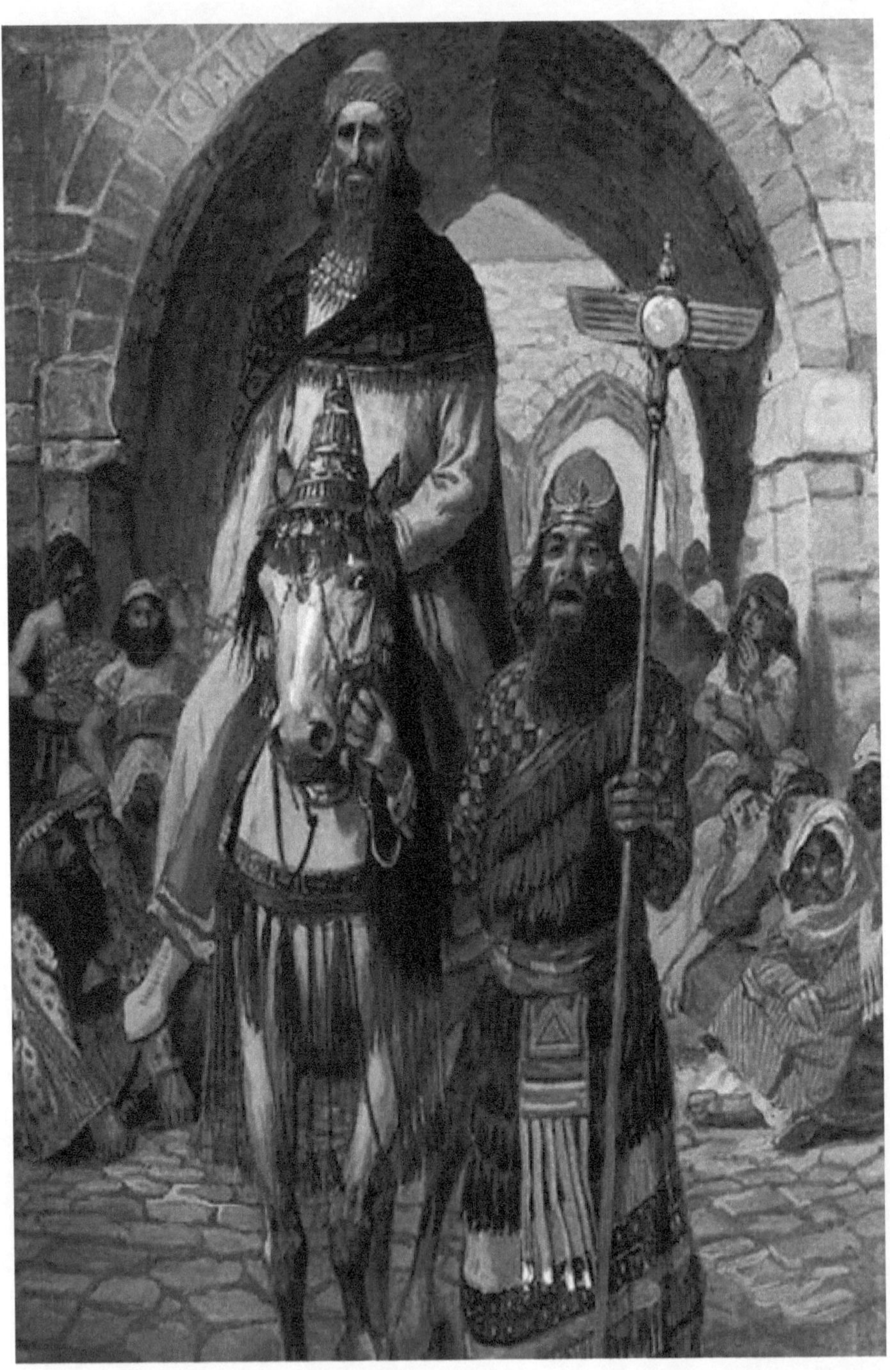

Later on, the king makes Mor′de·cai the second in command to himself. Mor′de·cai then ensures that a new law was made that permits the Israelites to fight for their lives on the day they're presupposed to be killed. Because Mor′de·cai is such an essential man now, many humans assist the Israelites, and they were delivered from the hands of their enemies.

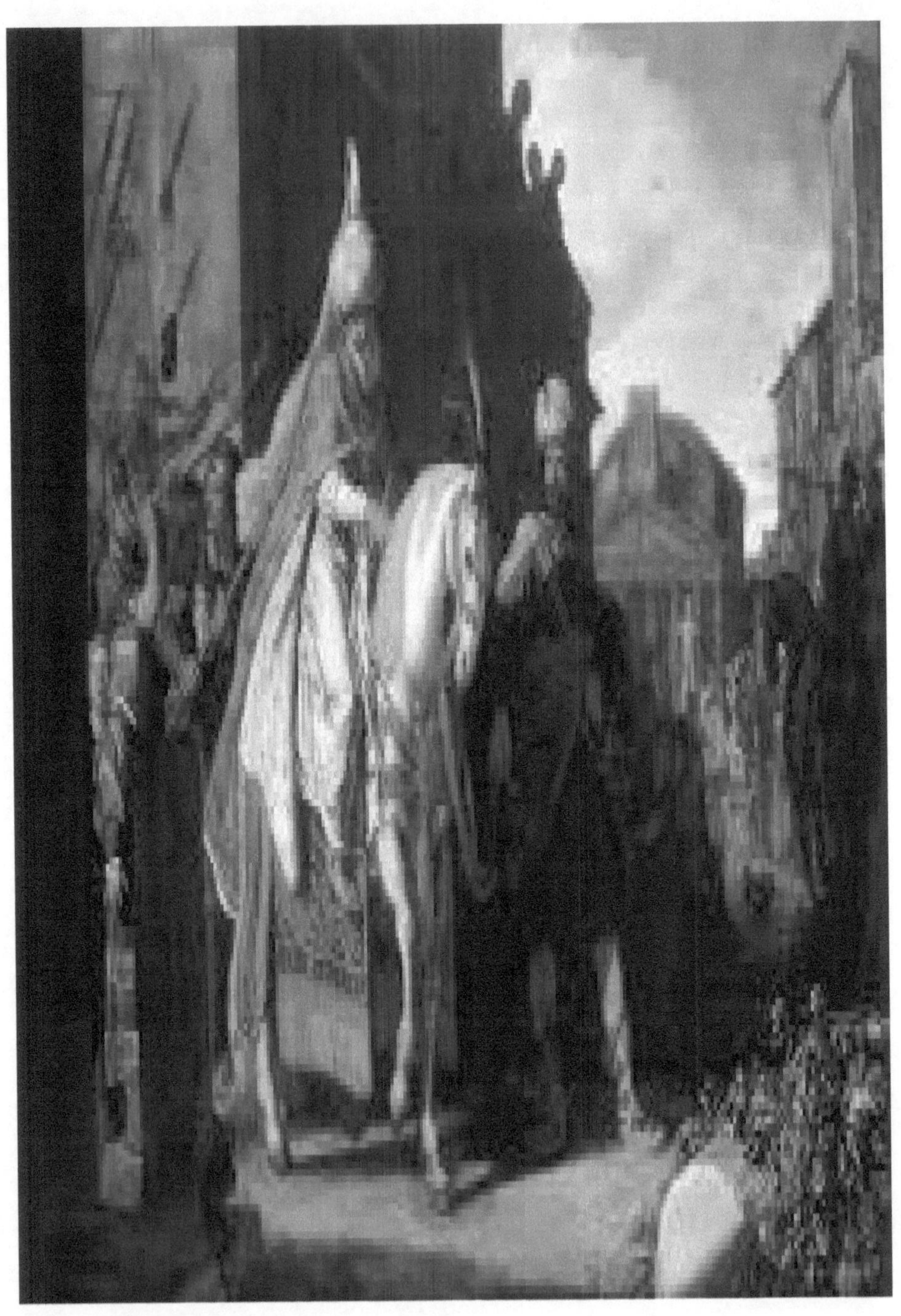

The rejected was celenrated by those who reject him

Esther10: 3 "Mordecai the jew became next in rank to king Ahasuerus, distinguished amidst the jews, and held in high esteem through his many fellow jews, due to the fact that he worked for the best of his human beings and spoke up for the welfare of all of the jews."

This must be mordecai's defining scripture – this has to be the verse that explains why he is who he is! Why he changed into the chief he changed into…

Permit's care deeply

Permit's be described by our love

Permit's be described by our situation for

the welfare of others.

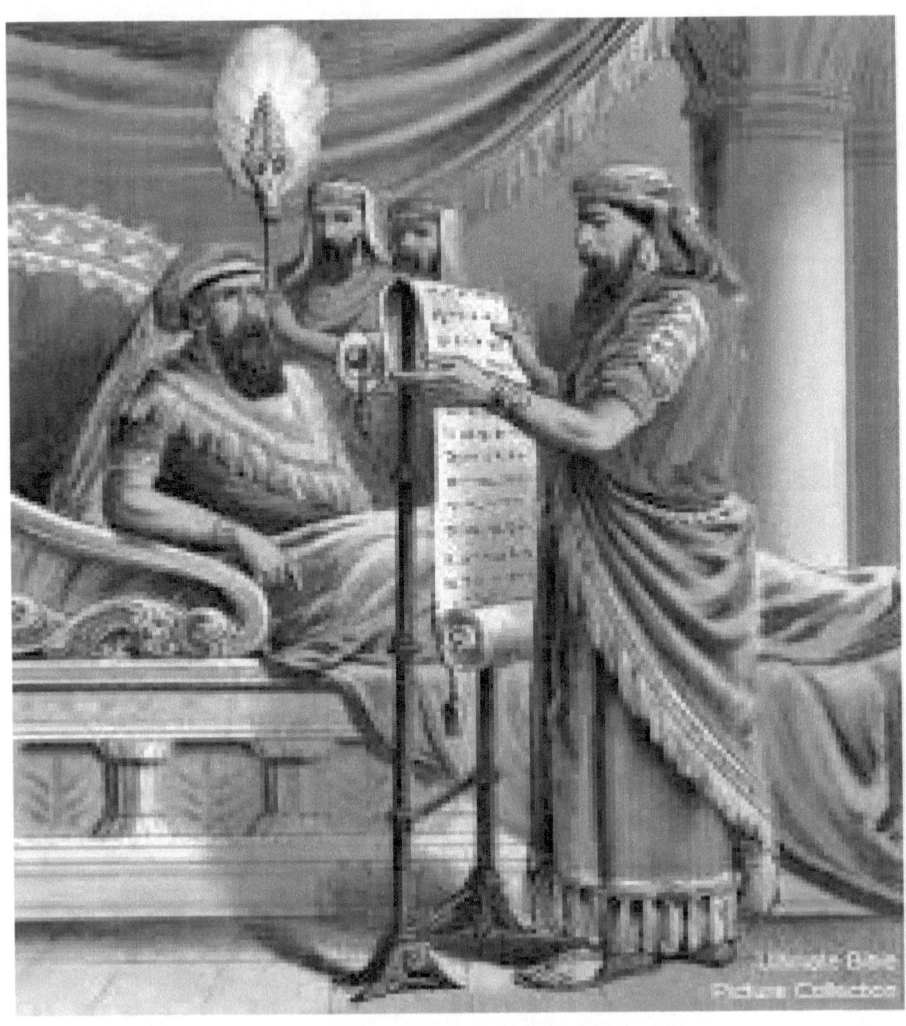

Let's be known for our right deeds

About the Author

Sunday O. Aduragbemi studied at the University of Columbia where he received his BA certificate in bology. He was a medical practitioner who had always been interested in the safety and maintenance of the human health and was able to effectively carry out the task therein, zealeously and to the best of his ability. He has devoted himself to the study of human physiology and botany and has been meeting the medical demand of the members of his society. With the help of God, he has help countless persons discover who they are and

what they stand to achieve if they can be

diligent and committed to whatever they do.

Acknowledgments

All glory to God Almighty who has made it possible to successfully complete the collation of this Bible story through the help and leadings of the Holy Spirit. And my appreciation also goes to my family members, friends, relatives, well wishers, who has in one way or the other been part of this successful work. Without you all who has kept me going through your advice, encouragement and words of challenge, this might not be successful. May God

bless you all? Amen.

THANKS FOR READING